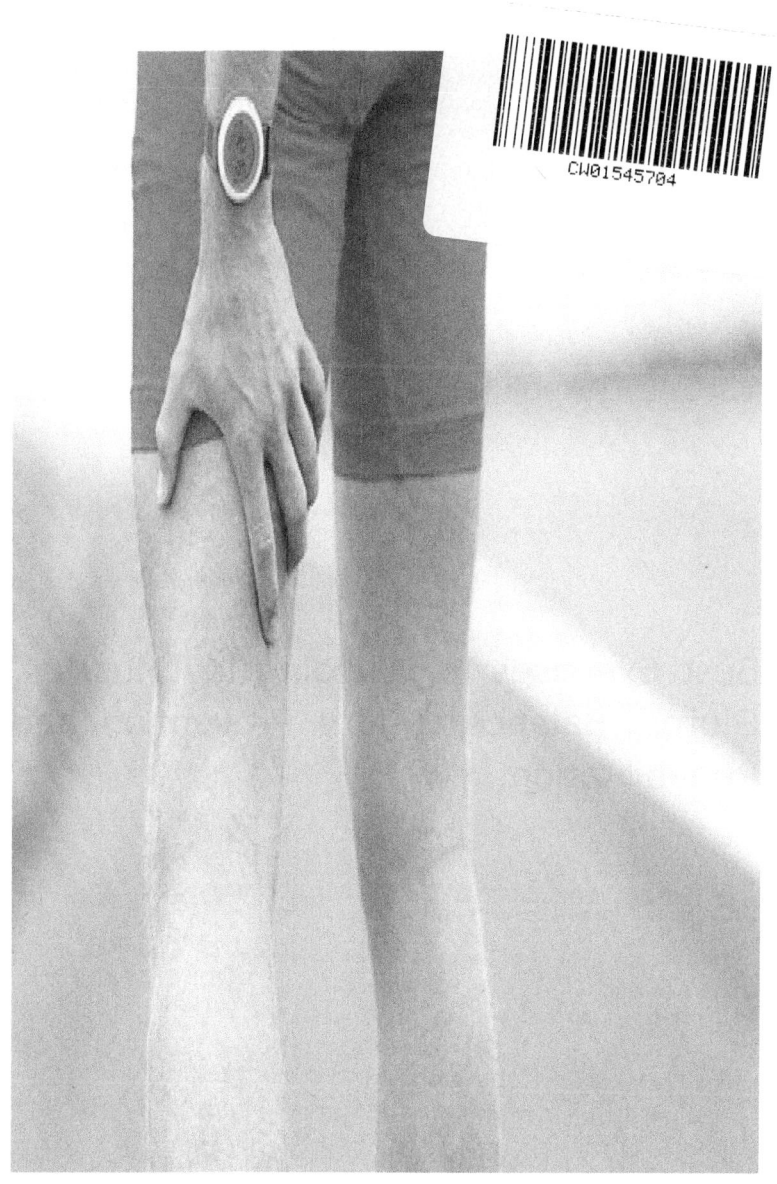

30 BEST LEG STRENGTHENING EXERCISES

Best Exercises for Building leg Muscles, Glutes, Balance, Injury Prevention and Rehabilitation.

CHARLINE GRIMMY

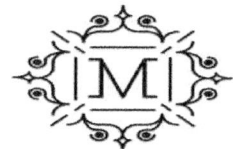

Copyright 2021 Morgan.

This book is subject to copyright policy. All rights are reserved, whether the entire or component of the material, particularly the right of transformation, reprinting, recycling illustration, broadcasting, duplicating on microfilm, or in any other way. No part or even the whole of this book or contents may be produced or even transmitted or reproduced in any way, be it electronic or paper form or by any means, electronic or mechanical, also include recording or by any information storage or retrieval system, without prior written permission the copyright owner, *Morgan LTD*

TABLE OF CONTENTS

LEG STRENGTHENING EXERCISES ..2
INTRODUCTION 7
PART 1: REASONS, BENEFITS, AND CAUTIONS..9
REASONS WHY YOU SHOULD NOT SKIP LEG STRENGTHENING EXERCISES 10
SKIPPING LEG STRENGTHENING EXERCISES......................................13
BENEFITS OF LEG WORKOUTS 15
PART 2: LEG MUSCLES AND STRUCTURES 18
FRONT THIGH MUSCLES...................19
HAMSTRINGS MUSCLES 22
CALF MUSCLES 23
PART 3: EFFECT OF NOT WORKING ON YOUR LEGS 26
FITNESS EXPERT IDEAS: 28

PART 4: BEST LEG STRENGTHENING EXERCISES 29
ALTERNATING KNEE LIFT 30
PLANK LEG LIFTS 32
SINGLE STRAIGHT LEG RAISE...........33
SQUATS WORKOUT 35
STABILITY BALL KNEE TUCKS 37
BANDED LATERAL WALK...................39
LUNGES WORKOUT.........................40
SUMO DEADLIFT 42
LATERAL LUNGE WITH BALANCE 44
CALF RAISE 45
SQUAT WITH HEEL RAISE.................47
BULGARIAN SPLIT SQUAT.................49
SIDE HIP RAISE 50
LATERAL STEP-OUT SQUAT...............51
KNEE EXTENSION............................53
CURTSY LUNGE 54
KNEE CURLS..................................56
LEG EXTENSIONS 58
LEG BALANCE 59

ISOMETRIC CALF RAISE 61
DUCK WALK...................................... 63
PISTOL SQUAT 65
MINI-BAND CLAMSHELLS 67
BANDED GLUTE BRIDGE................... 69

INTRODUCTION

Legs are part of our lower body that plays a major role in our daily activities. The legs are the main part of the body that keeps you all day long Walking, jumping, running and balancing. They also provide support and flexibility for your body and allow you to participate in most regular activities.

You are not only working the primary muscles in your legs when you undertake these leg strengthening exercises and routines. You will also strengthen your core, enhance your balance, as well as improve your strength.

In this book, we have discussed various leg strengthening exercises that will enhance your leg muscles, balance, strength, injury preventions and rehabilitations. These exercises target all parts of the legs including the knees, calves and thighs.

Strong legs do more than just look good. Even the most basic daily activities such as walking, need leg strength. This simply means that including leg workouts in your daily routine is essential to your overall fitness.

PART 1: REASONS, BENEFITS, AND CAUTIONS

Leg strengthening exercises are important for building leg muscles but they are sometimes overlooked in favor of upper-body training. Instead, it is better to stick to exercise routine that promotes a healthy body, which involves a strong solid base of both the upper and lower body.

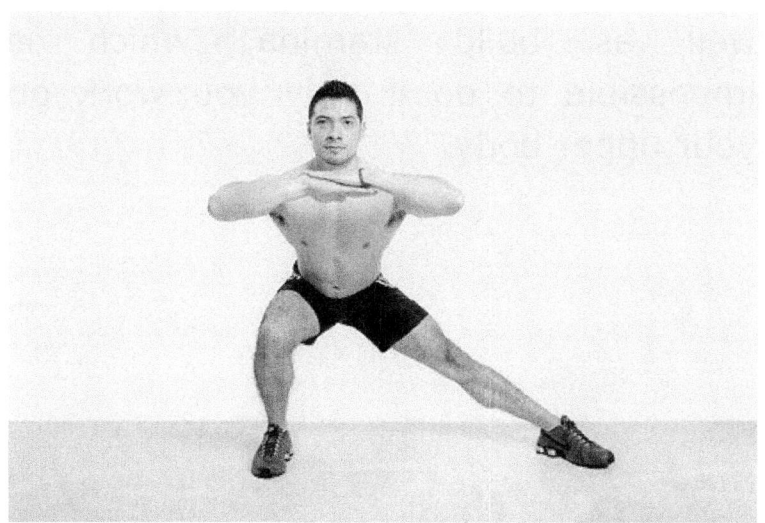

REASONS WHY YOU SHOULD NOT SKIP LEG STRENGTHENING EXERCISES

Leg workouts should be done regularly because some of the large muscles are found in our legs and they are vital parts of our total body. Furthermore, your body will have an easier time adapting to the workouts and developing excellent flexibility and stamina that will help you achieve your fitness objectives. Strong leg muscles help you to keep your body balanced as well as build stamina, which is impossible to do if only you work on your upper body.

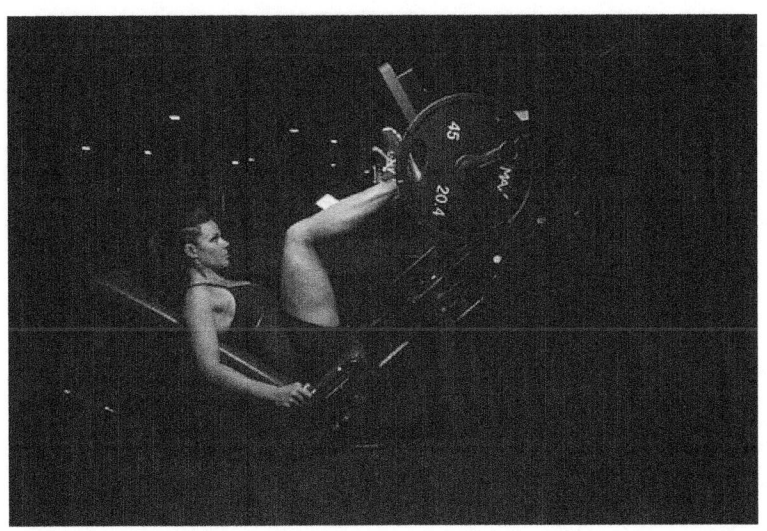

Workouts like deadlifts, squats, as well as lunges help you to enhance and increase athletic efficiency by working your glutes, quadriceps, as well as hamstrings. Avoid overworking your quads by combining glutes and hamstrings into your routine exercise program. The muscle of the lower body provides a strong and stable balance.

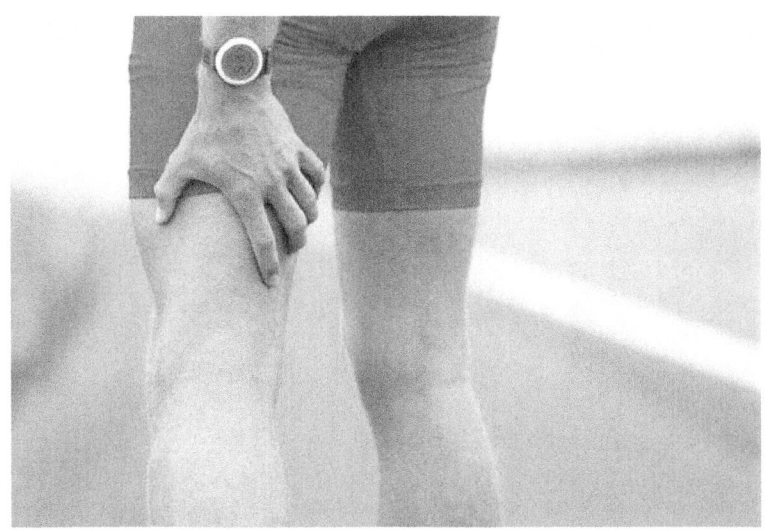

By lowering your lower body towards the ground, you may generate resistance that flows up through your core as well as your upper body. All sorts of motions, including upper-body activities like throwing, batting, and reaching an object at the top all rely on lower-body strength and stability. If the lower body is weak you may experience accidents and injuries.

SKIPPING LEG STRENGTHENING EXERCISES

Unless you have an injury, It's possible that you will be exhausted or have a further injury if you continue or engage in these exercises.

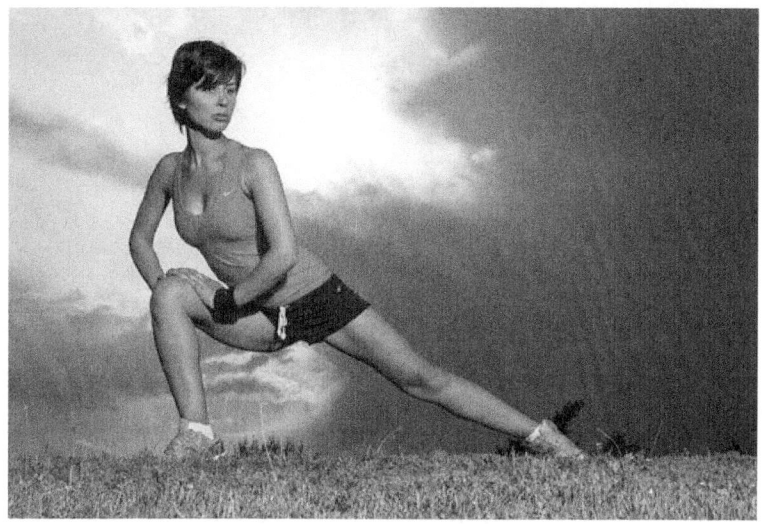

It is best to consult your doctor for advice on whether you should continue the exercises or not.

If you have chest tightness or congestion, exhaustion, or severe muscular discomfort these are some signs that you should take a rest.

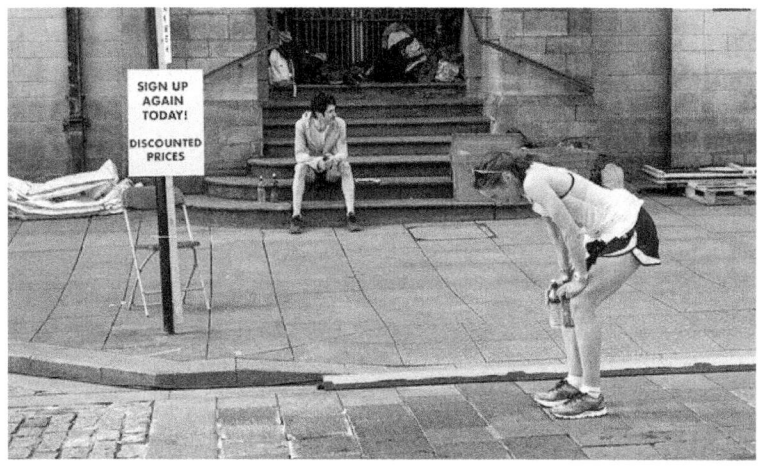

When you are ill, don't push yourself when you feel uncomfortable this may slow down your recuperation or create more injury. Therefore you need to take it easy. Taking some time off and it will aid in your recuperation.

BENEFITS OF LEG WORKOUTS

Strengthening your legs involves all of your body's major muscle groups, which aids in overall performance as well as promotes healthy body movement.

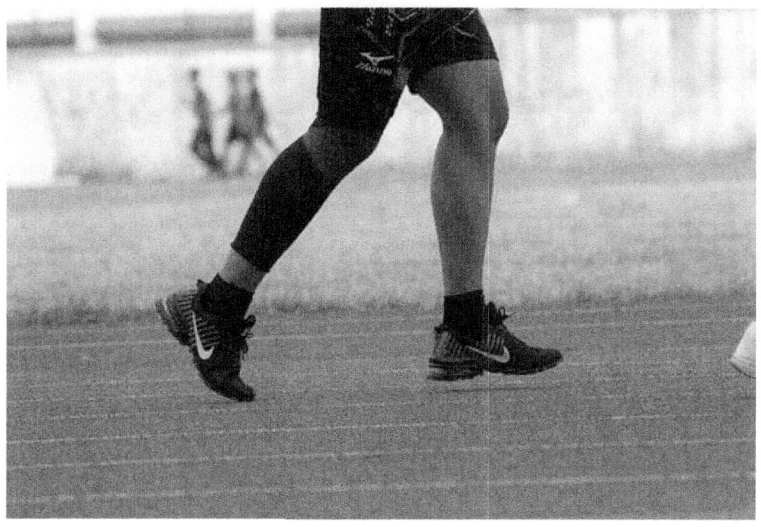

A strong lower body will also aid in the prevention of injury as well as the management of chronic illnesses and arthritis, heart disease, including diabetes.

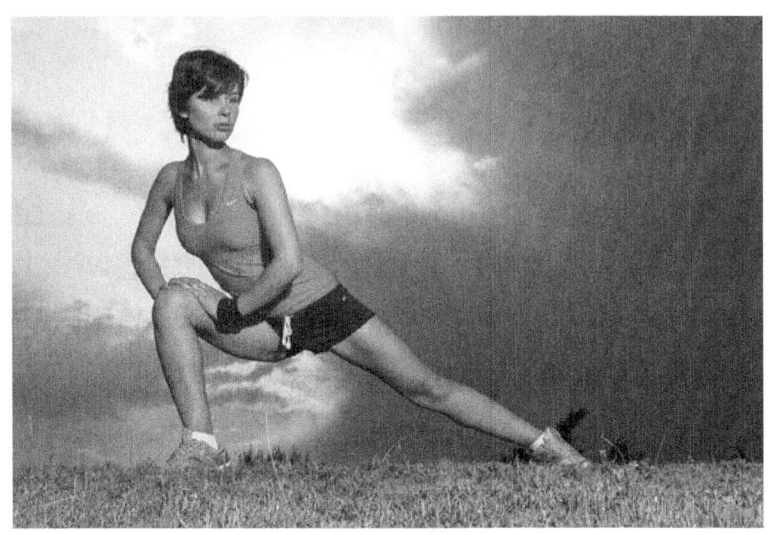

The followings are the benefits of leg strengthening exercises:

- It assists in improving hormones like testosterone, human growth hormones as well as cortisol.
- Strengthen balance and prevent falling.
- It engages the core muscles.
- It builds and strengthens the leg muscles.
- Improve tone and sculpt legs.
- Burning of fat and lead to weight loss.
- It improves the range of motions.

- It reduces joint pains
- Strengthen and boost bones.
- Improve stability, posture and movement.
- Injury preventions and rehabilitations

PART 2: LEG MUSCLES AND STRUCTURES

Most of the muscles in our lower body mostly the legs are found to be long muscles, They extend across a considerable distance. These muscles contract as well as relax, causing skeletal bones to move, allowing movement and stability to occur. Smaller muscles assist bigger muscles in stabilizing joints, rotating joints, balance, and performing other fine-tuned motions.

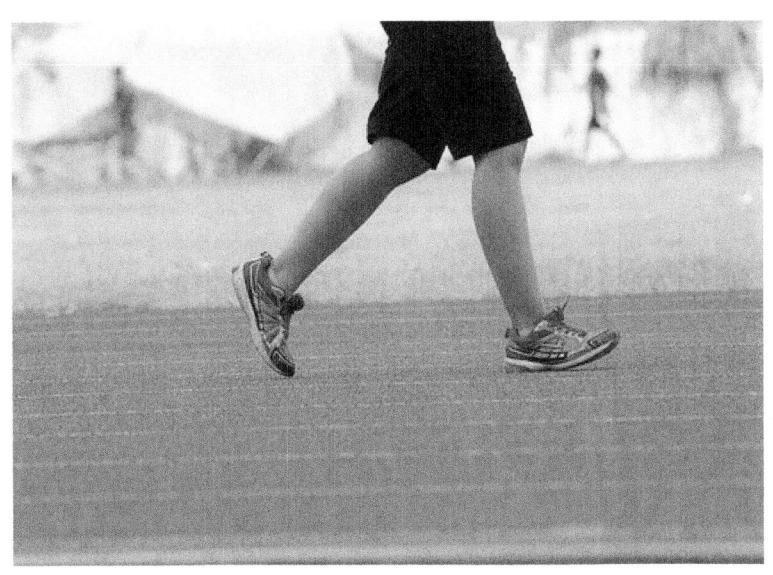

FRONT THIGH MUSCLES

The thigh, as well as the calf, contain the major muscle masses that are found in the leg. Quadriceps are found to be one of the strongest as well as the leanest muscles in our body.

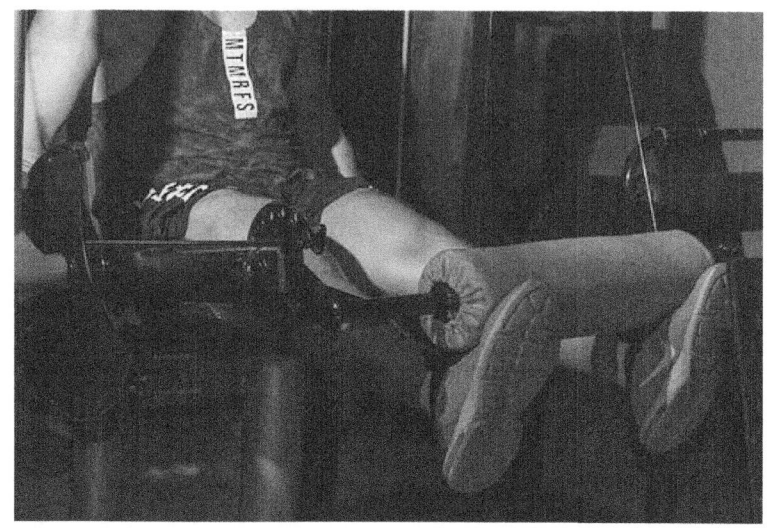

Extensors are one of the muscles found at the front thigh whose most function is to lengthen the leg straight.

They are:

The Rectus Femoris	These muscles are found at the kneecap of the major quadriceps muscles. This muscle has little effect on the flexion of the knee.
Vastus Intermedius	They are found in between the vastus lateralis as well as

	the vastus medialis at the front side of the femur.
Vastus Medialis	This teardrop muscle shape of the inner part of the thigh is found in the femur as well as down to the innermost part of the border of the kneecap.
Vastus lateralis	This is the biggest quadriceps muscle on the thigh. It runs from the apex of the femur to the patella (kneecap).

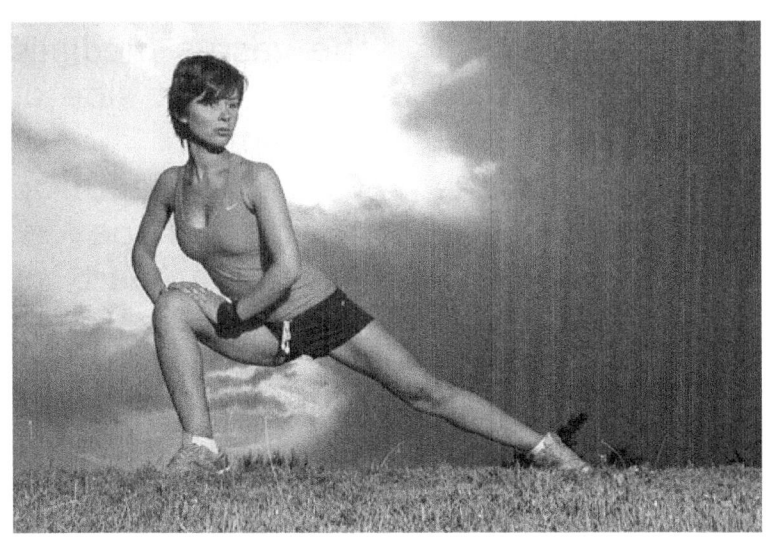

HAMSTRINGS MUSCLES

The hamstrings are found at the thighs mostly at the back, which affects the hip as well as knee movement. They begin from the gluteus maximus found behind the hipbone as well as at the knee it is attached to the tibia.

Biceps femoris	The knee is flexed by this lengthy muscle. It starts in the thigh and to the fibula's head close to the knee.
Semimembranosus	From the pelvis to the tibia, this

	lengthy muscle runs. It assists rotate the tibia by extending the thigh, flexing the knee, and also extending the thigh.
Semitendinosus	This muscle also flexes the knee as well as extends the thigh.

CALF MUSCLES

The calf muscles are important aspects of ankle, foot, as well as toe mobility.

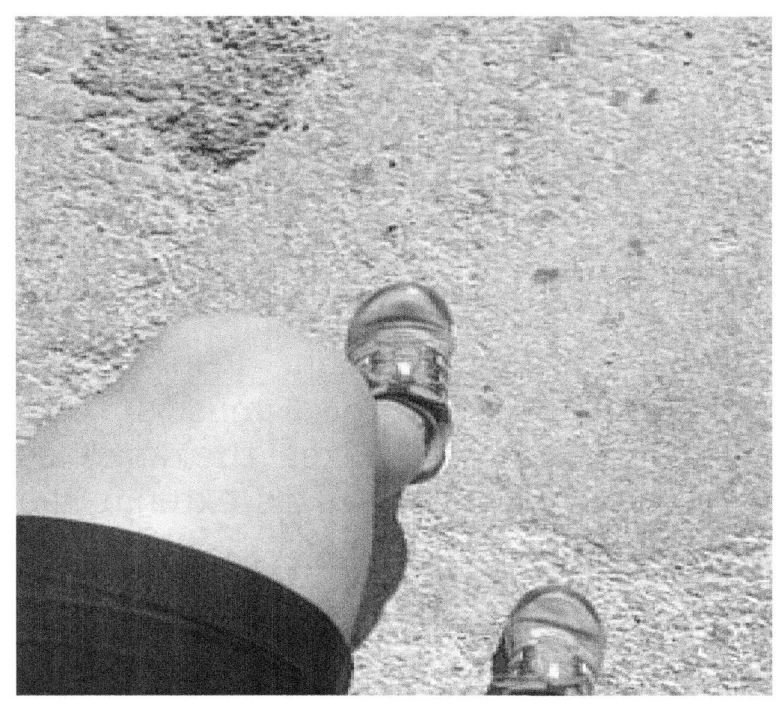

The following are some of the primary calf muscles:

Plantaris	About 10% of people lack this small thin muscle. Its role is superseded by the gastrocnemius muscle.
Soleus	These muscles are connected from the backside of the knee down to the heel. It plays a major part in

	walking as well as standing.
Gastrocnemius	It links to the heel and also the leg major muscles. It allows the foot, ankle, as well as knee to bend and extend.

PART 3: EFFECT OF NOT WORKING ON YOUR LEGS

If you don't strengthen your leg muscles, you won't be able to build your balance and resistance against any falls for all of your activities. Stamina and balance will provide you with increased stability, improving your mobility, range of motion, as well as coordination.

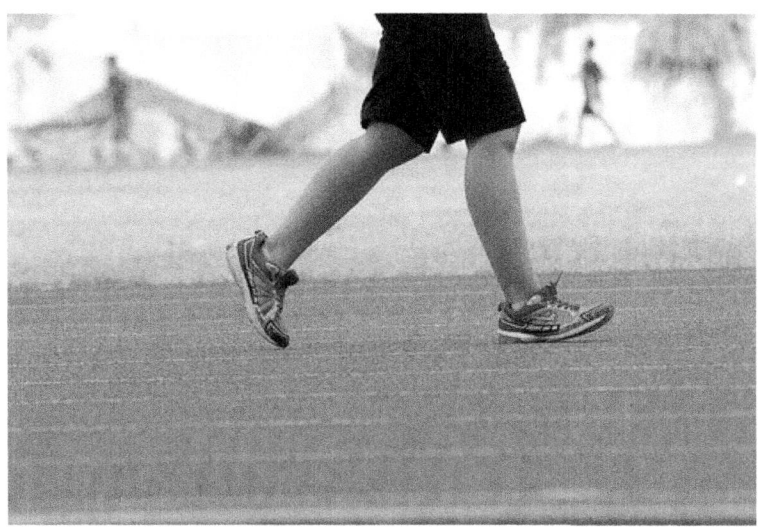

You are not only working the primary muscles in your legs when you undertake these leg exercises. You also strengthen your core, enhance your balance, as well as refine your grip strength, all of which pay off in the long term.

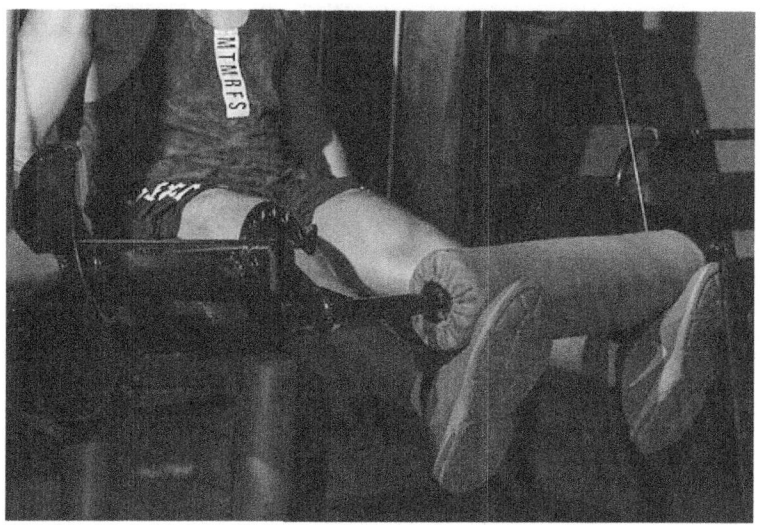

Your muscle might decrease with time while your fat cell grows. You may look and feel less fit and muscular as a result of this. If you only work your upper body and ignore your legs or lower body you may not be able to resist any heavy or force that will require stamina.

FITNESS EXPERT IDEAS:

A fitness coach can assist you in developing a well-balanced fitness program that combines leg exercises as well as cardiovascular, balance and also flexibility training.

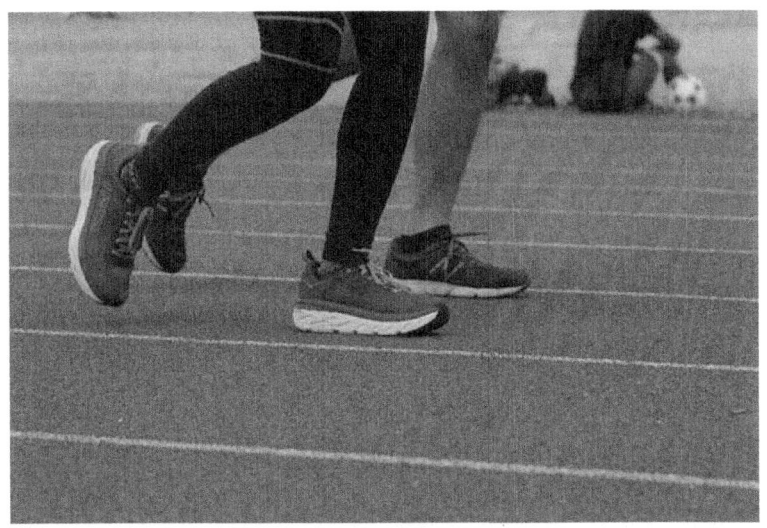

If you are new to fitness or want to alter up your current routine, talk to a fitness instructor about your leg training objectives. Even if you already have a training routine, a fitness professional can give you some new ideas to keep you fit.

PART 4: BEST LEG STRENGTHENING EXERCISES

Leg workouts engage the muscles around your legs, so keeping them toned offers a lot of advantages. Your leg strength enhances your metabolism while improving strength and balance.

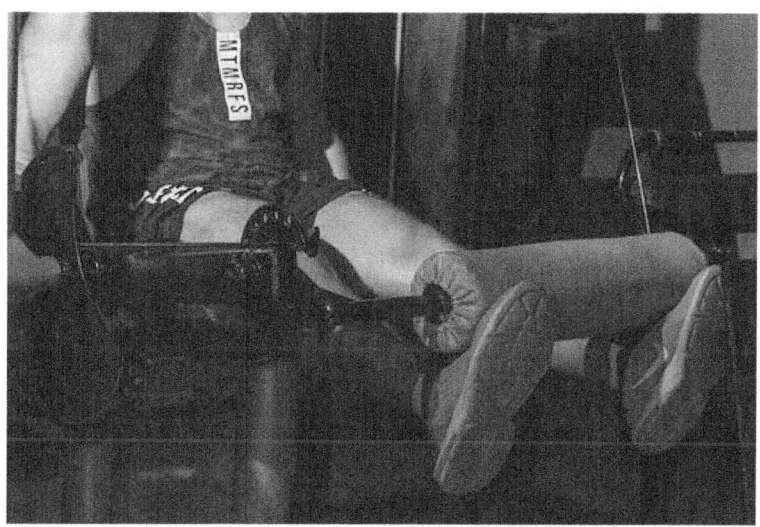

The followings are the best leg strengthening exercises that will build your muscles, strength, balance, and stability.

ALTERNATING KNEE LIFT

BENEFIT:

This exercise helps to build your muscle, balance, stability and range of motion. It is also suitable for injury recovery and rehabilitation.

TARGET:

Quads, Hamstrings and Glutes.

PROCEDURE:

- Start by standing upright with your feet.
- Raise your knee right leg above the floor level to your hip level while your left leg is on the floor for support.
- Return your right leg to the ground while you immediately raise your

left leg above the floor. Do this at pace.
- Repeat 15-20 times, 2-3 sets.

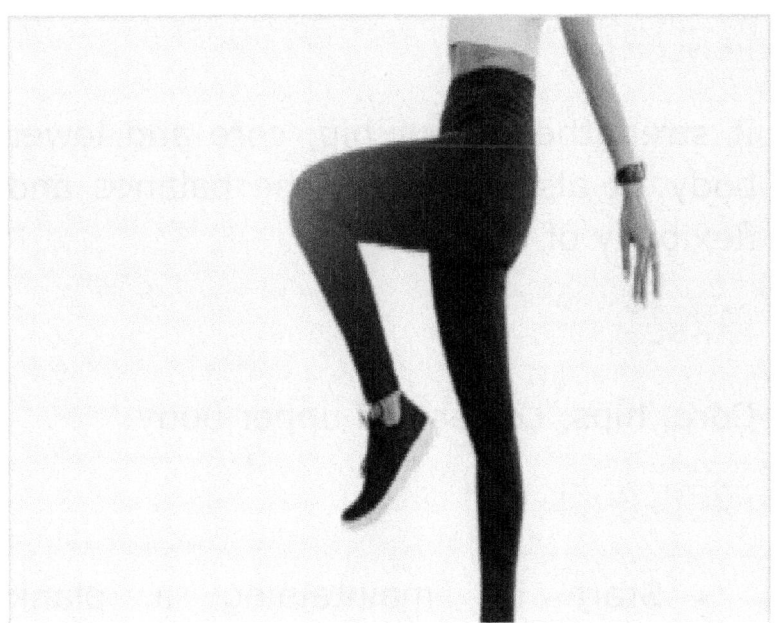

PLANK LEG LIFTS

BENEFIT:

It strengthens your hip, core and lower body. It also improves the balance and flexibility of the legs.

TARGET:

Core, hips, Lower and upper body.

PROCEDURE:

- Start by maintaining a plank position while your both palms are on the floor.
- Raise one of your leg from the back above your buttocks from your hip joint.
- Gently and gradually return your leg slowly to the floor level with the other leg and do the same with the other leg. Rep 5-7 times and sets 2-3.

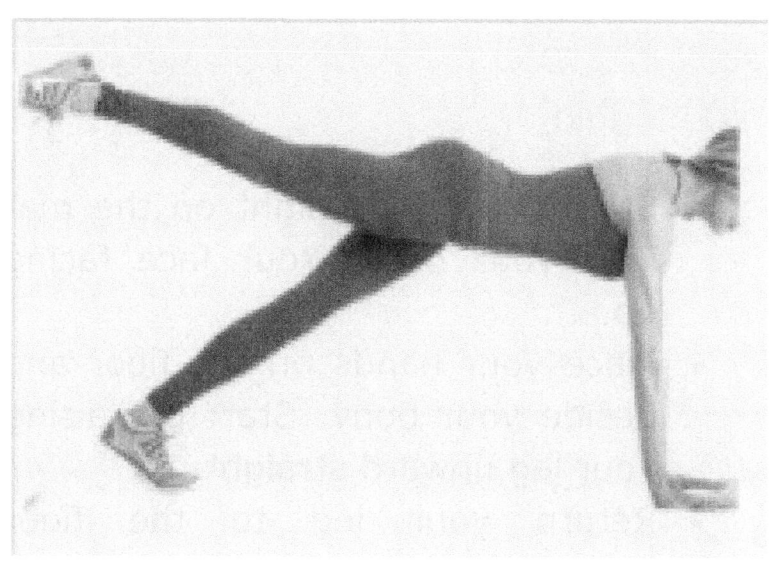

SINGLE STRAIGHT LEG RAISE

BENEFIT:

It helps to strengthen the hips, joints and also improve balance and flexibility. Best for injury recovery, prevention and rehabilitation.

TARGET:

Upper legs, hips and butt.

PROCEDURE:

- Start by lying straight on the mat with your back. Your face facing up.
- Place your hands on the floor and beside your body. Start by raising your leg upward straight.
- Return your leg to the floor immediately raise the other leg. continue at pace.
- Rep 5-10. Sets 2-5.

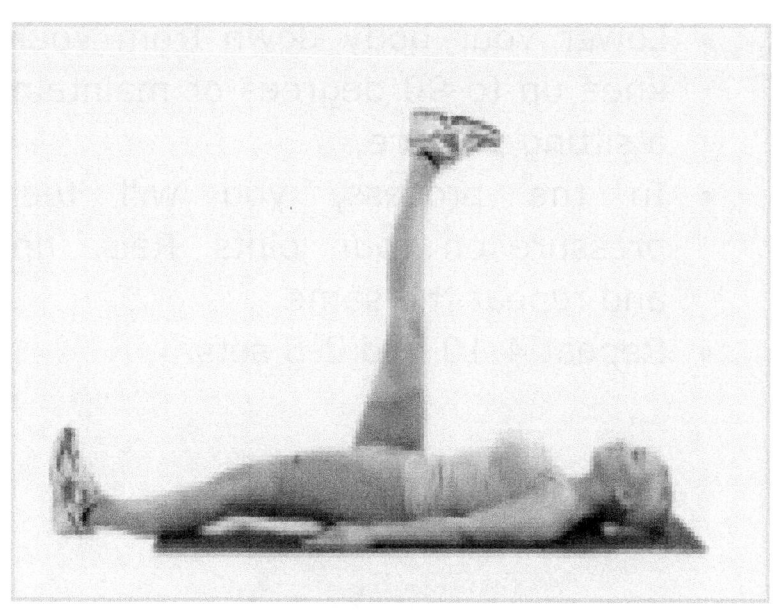

SQUATS WORKOUT

BENEFIT::

Strengthen the knee joints, improve or build muscles and increase stability.

TARGET:

Thighs, hips and knee joints

PROCEDURE:

- Firstly, stand upright with your feet on the floor.

- Lower your body down from your knee up to 90 degrees or maintain a sitting posture.
- In the process, you will feel pressure on your joints. Raise up and repeat the same.
- Repeat 4-10 and 2-5 sets.

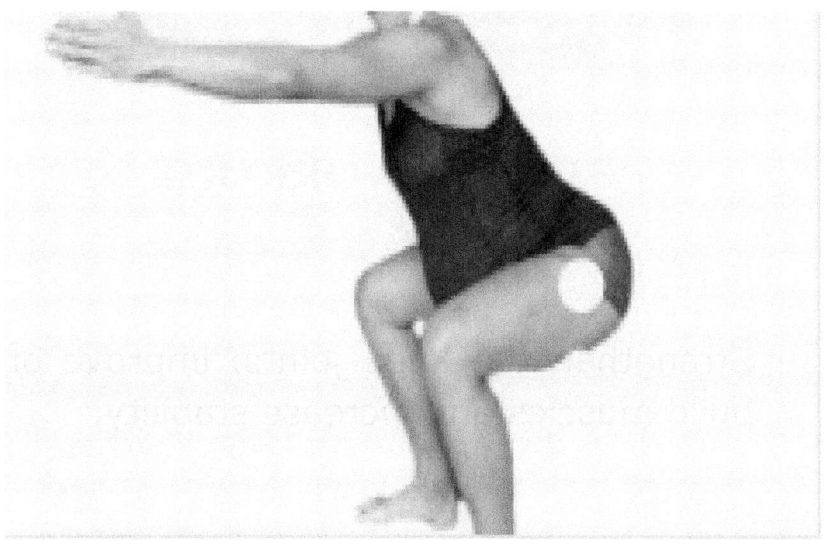

STABILITY BALL KNEE TUCKS

BENEFITS:

It helps to strengthen the knee joints as well as the flexibility of your legs. Exercise for injury recovery, prevention and rehabilitation.

TARGET:

Knee joints, hips and toes.

PROCEDURE:

- Start by performing a plank pose but this time around you will need a stability ball to place your both legs on.
- Ensure that your legs are properly placed on the ball and your palms placed on the floor for support.

- Roll the ball forward towards your hips and your knee bent to the chest.
- Return by rolling the ball backward and your leg fully stretches.
- Repeat up to 3-10 times and set 2-4.

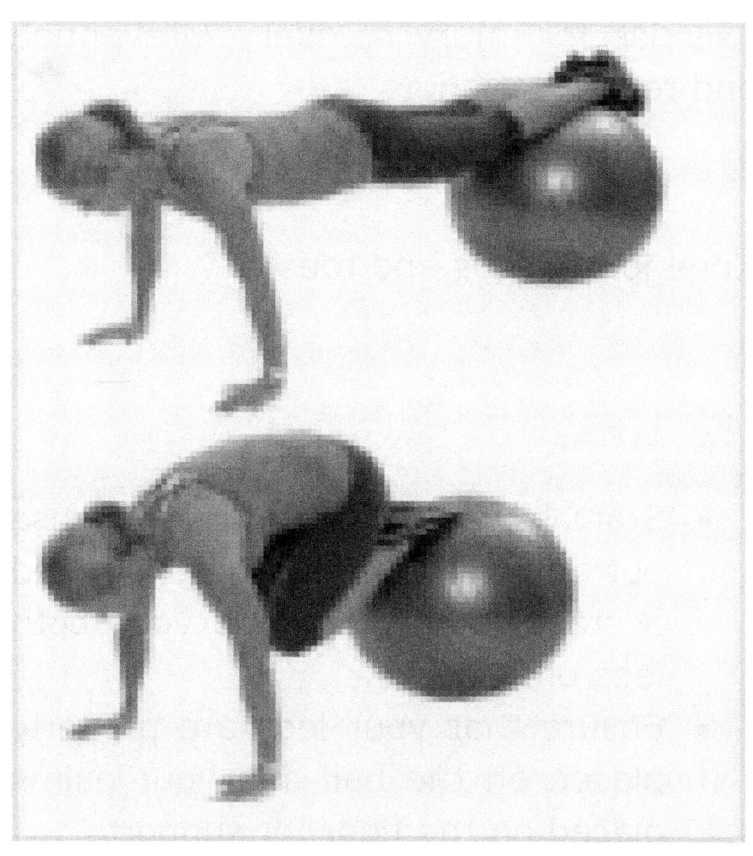

BANDED LATERAL WALK

BENEFIT:

It Improves range of motion, flexibility and stability. Exercise for injury recovery, prevention and rehabilitation.

TARGET:

This exercise warm up your glutes as well as target the glute medius muscles, which are typically overlooked.

PROCEDURE:

- Stand upright with your feet apart as well as knees slightly bent. Place a small resistance band just a few inches above ankles.
- Step out to the side with your left foot first, then your right, keeping your core tight.
- That counts as one rep. Perform five to seven sets of 10 to 12 reps on each side, then take a 30- to

60-second break before moving on to the next exercise.

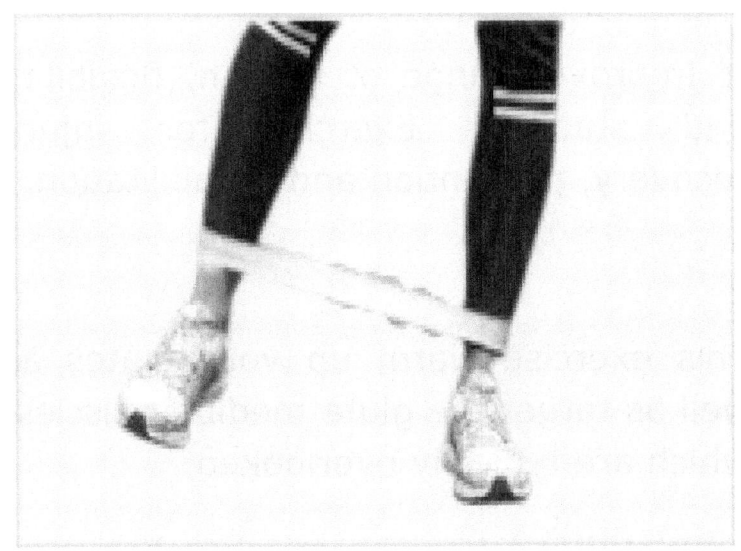

LUNGES WORKOUT

BENEFITS:

It strengthens the legs and joints, improves flexibility and stability.

TARGETS:

Calves, hamstrings, glutes and thighs.

PROCEDURE:

- Start by standing upright with your feet on the floor.
- Step forward with your right foot while dropping your back knee down toward the floor.
- Push off your back foot to move back to your stand position.
- Repeat the same with the other leg.

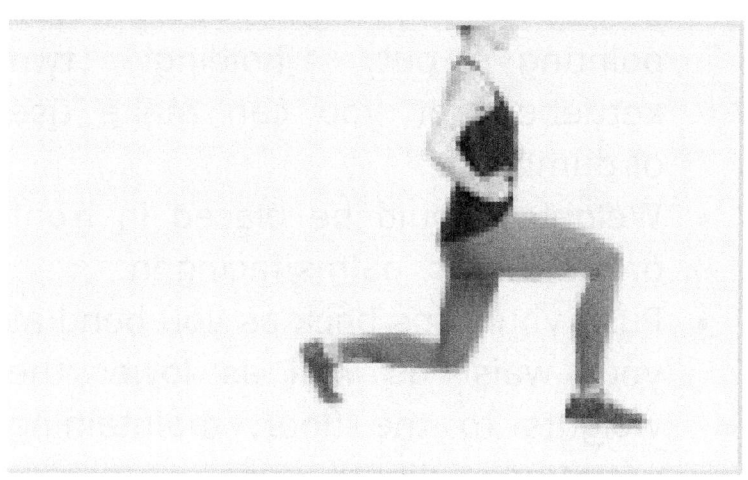

SUMO DEADLIFT

BENEFIT:

Build muscles, Balance and prevent falls.

TARGET:

Hamstrings, thighs and back.

PROCEDURE:

- Pose with your feet slightly wide and your hip-width apart, toes pointing out, holding two kettlebells or you can make use of dumbbells.
- Weights should be placed in front of the thighs, palms facing in.
- Push your hips back as you bend at your waist as well as lower the weights to the floor, maintaining your knees slightly bent.

- Return to a standing position by squeezing or tightening your glutes. That counts as one rep.
- Perform three or four sets of ten to twelve reps, then rest for 40 to 60 seconds before moving on to the next exercise.

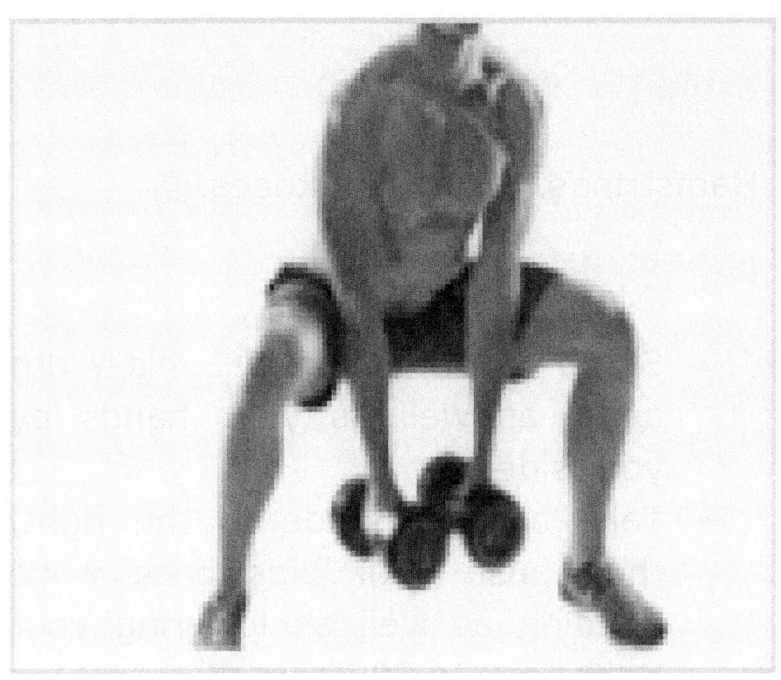

LATERAL LUNGE WITH BALANCE

BENEFITS:

It improves stability, flexibility and range of motion. Exercise for injury recovery, prevention and rehabilitation.

TARGET:

Hamstrings, thighs and knees.

PROCEDURE:

- Stand with your feet hip-width apart as well as your hands by your sides.
- Take a large stride to the right, then push your hips back while bending as well as lowering your right knee to 90 degrees.
- Return to a standing position by raising your knee and bringing it toward your chest with your arms.
- That counts as one rep. Perform three or four sets of ten to twelve

reps on each side, then rest for 30 to 60 seconds before moving on to the next exercise.

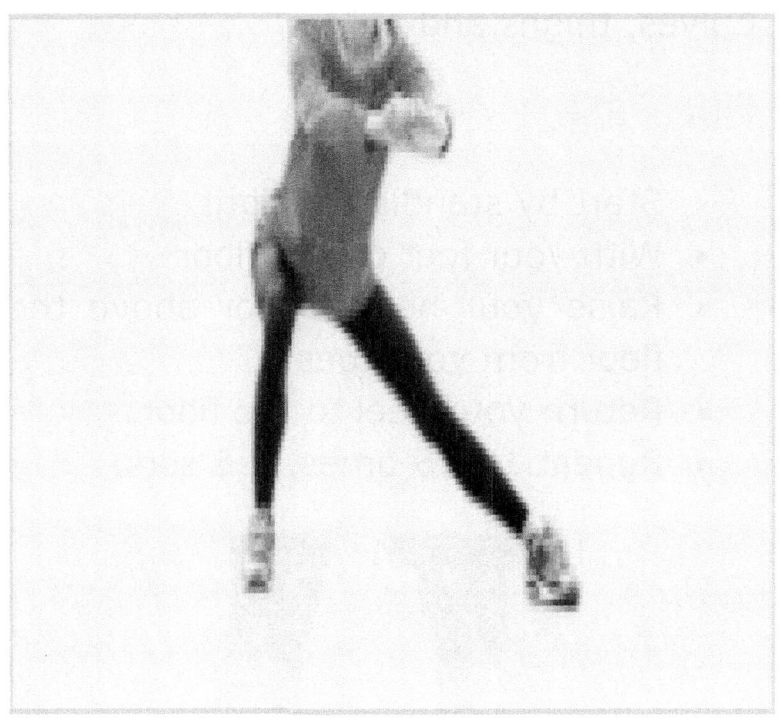

CALF RAISE

BENEFITS:

Strengthen your calves, improve balance and build muscles.

TARGETS:

Calves, thighs and ankles.

PROCEDURE:

- Start by standing upright.
- With your feet on the floor.
- Raise your heels up or above the floor from your toes.
- Return your heel to the floor.
- Repeat 10-15 times, 3-5 sets.

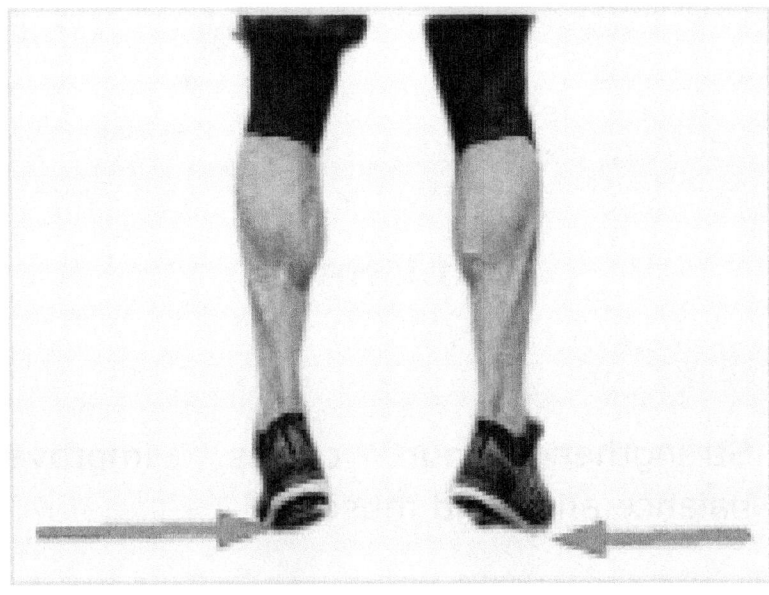

SQUAT WITH HEEL RAISE

BENEFITS:

It helps to strengthen the knee joints, improve balance and flexibility. Exercise for injury recovery, prevention and rehabilitation.

TARGET:

Target your calves.

PROCEDURE:

- Stand with your toes on the floor. ensure that it turned out slightly as well as your heels wider than shoulder apart.
- Bend your knees, stretch your hips back, as well as squat.
- Drop your arms between your legs. Then, when you rise up, circle your arms out to the sides.

- Lift your arms straight up and push up your toes. That counts as one rep. Perform 3 or 4 sets of ten to twelve reps, then rest for 30 to 60 seconds before moving on to the next exercise.

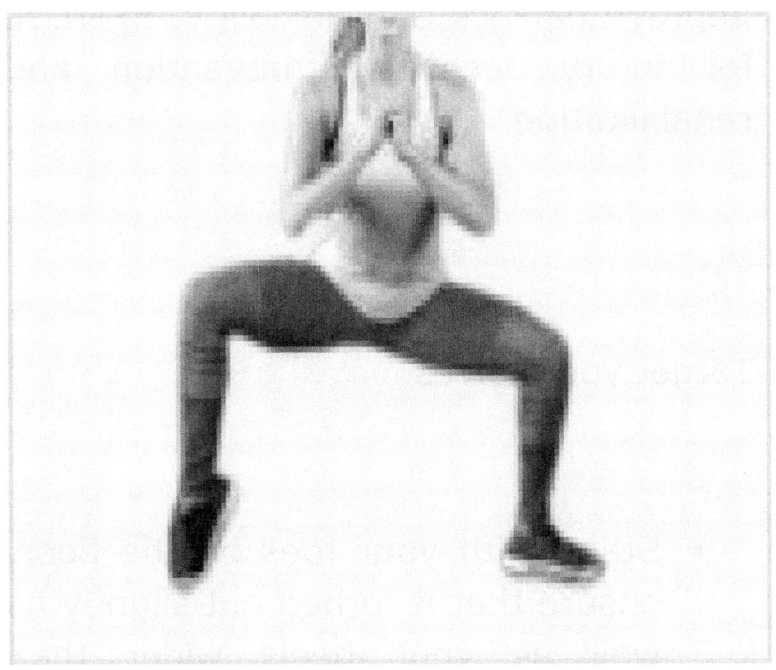

BULGARIAN SPLIT SQUAT

BENEFIT:

Strengthen the muscles, Hips joint flexibility and also improve your balance. Injury preventions and rehabilitations.

TARGET:

Hips, Glutes and foot joints.

PROCEDURE:

- Begin by standing two feet on the floor in front of a step with a weight in each hand. Place your left foot on the step as well as extend your left leg back.
- Maintain shoulders back as well as chest up as you bend knees to

lower body as far as you can (or until knee hovers just above the floor).
- Return to the start by pausing and pressing through the right heel. That counts as one rep. Perform 3 or 4 sets of ten to twelve reps on each side, then rest for thirty to sixty seconds before moving on to the next exercise.

SIDE HIP RAISE

BENEFITS:

Strengthen the muscles, Hips joint flexibility and also improve your balance.

TARGET:

Glutes, Hips and Thighs.

PROCEDURE:

Start by lying on the floor sideward with your hand stretched toward the floor as well as your body raised above the floor. Hold on to the position for some time (10-60 seconds). Repeat the same with the other hand.

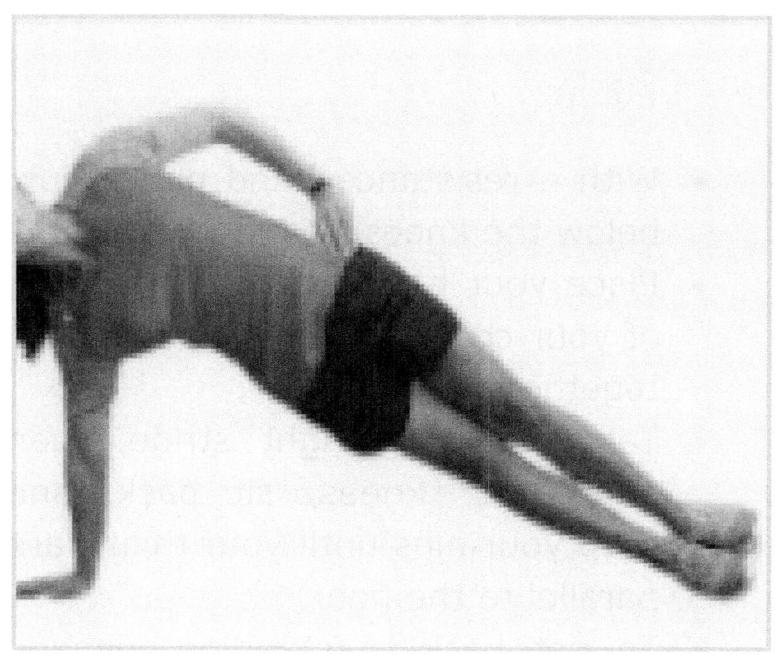

LATERAL STEP-OUT SQUAT

BENEFIT:

Strengthen the bone, Hips joint flexibility and also improve your balance. Injury preventions and rehabilitations.

TARGET:

Glutes, thighs and quads.

PROCEDURE:

- With a resistance band placed just below the knees, stand up straight.
- Place your hands right in the front of your chest as well as clasp them together.
- Take a strong right stride, then bend your knees, sit back, and drop your hips until your thighs are parallel to the floor.
- To get back to standing, engage your glutes as well as press up through your heels.
- That counts as one rep. Perform three or four sets of ten to twelve reps, then rest for thirty to sixty seconds before moving on to the next exercise.

KNEE EXTENSION

BENEFIT:

Strengthen the knee joints and improve the core muscles.

TARGET:

Quadriceps, knees and calves.

PROCEDURE:

- Start by sitting on a chair and your feet appropriately placed on the floor.
- Raise your leg upward above the floor. Your leg should be of equal level with your knee.
- Go back to the starting position. Repeat it with the left leg. Rep 10-15 times.

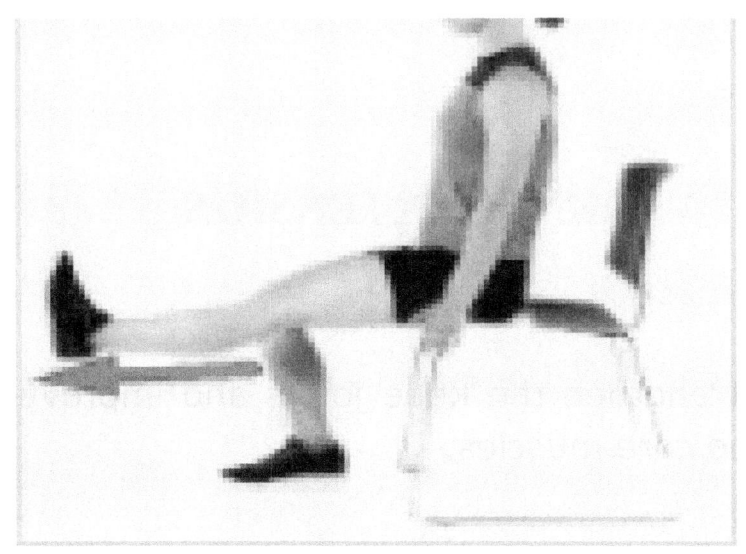

CURTSY LUNGE

BENEFITS:

Stronger lower body, improve stability and balance.

TARGET:

Thighs, quads and knees.

PROCEDURE:

- Hold strongly a dumbbell on both hands.

- Take a large stride back with your right leg while crossing it behind your left side.
- Lower your hips as well as bend your knees until your left thigh is closely equal with the floor.
- Maintain a straight torso and square hips and shoulders as feasible. Go back to the starting point.
- That counts as one rep. Perform five or six sets of ten to twelve reps on each side, then rest for thirty to sixty seconds before moving on to the next exercise.

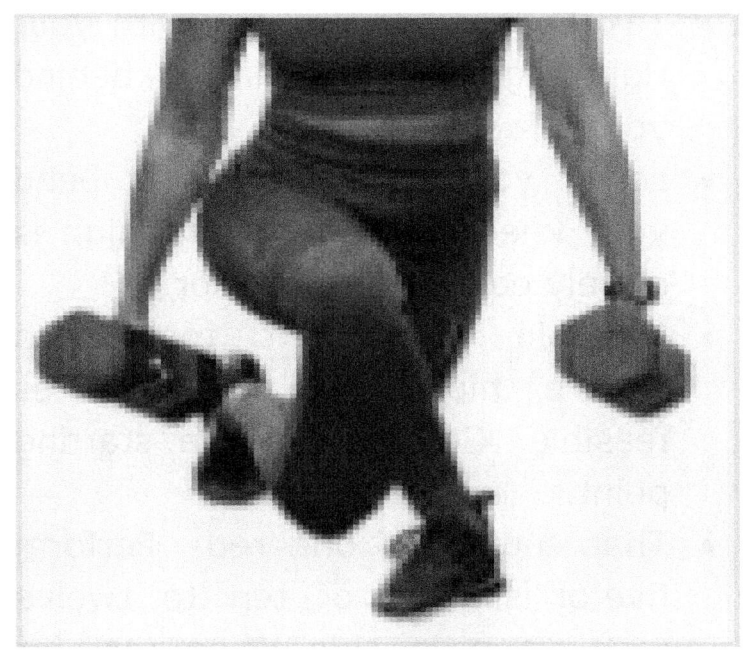

KNEE CURLS

BENEFIT:

Improve mobility, strengthen your core muscles around your legs and improve movement.

TARGET:

Hamstrings at your upper leg, knee joints and calves.

PROCEDURE:

- Start by standing upright.
- Lift your leg backward direction and use one of your hand to hold on to the foot of your leg while the other leg is properly placed on the floor for support.
- Stretch it upward. You will feel pressure around your knee joint.
- Rep 4-8, set 2-4.

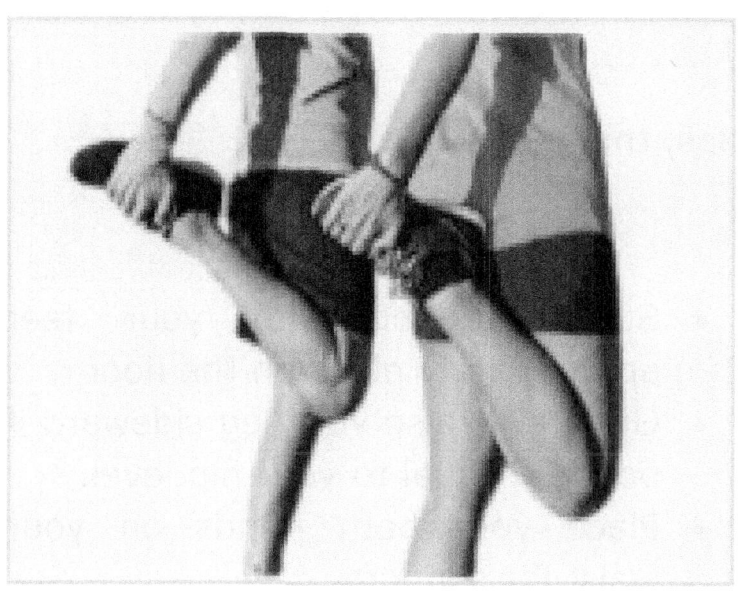

LEG EXTENSIONS

BENEFITS:

Leg extensions assist you to support your lower back by toning the muscles around your lower body. Injury prevents and rehabilitations.

TARGETS:

Hips, thighs and quadriceps.

PROCEDURE:

- Stand upright with your feet appropriately place on the floor.
- Gradually raise your leg sideward if possible equal to your hip level.
- Place your both hands on your waist for support.
- Return your leg to the floor and do the same with the other leg.

- Rep 8-15 and sets 2-4.

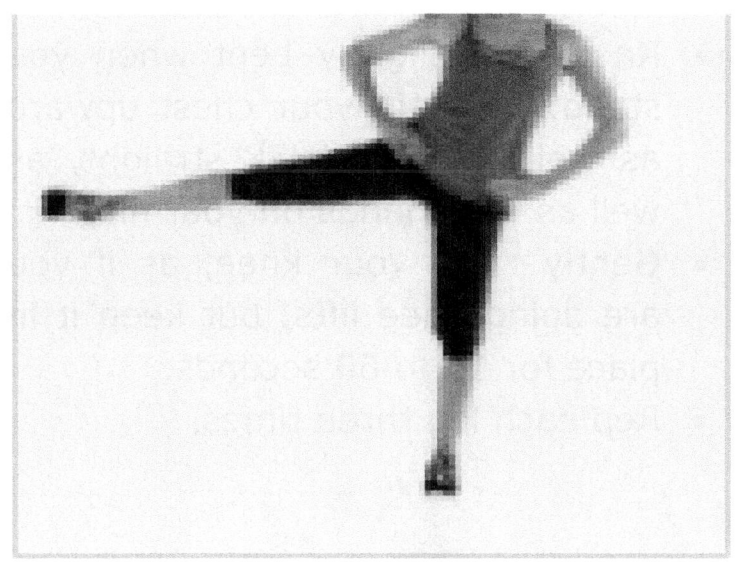

LEG BALANCE

BENEFIT:

Improve balance, flexibility and stability.

TARGET:

Hips, knee joints and hamstrings.

PROCEDURE:

- Knees are slightly bent when you stand. Maintain your chest upward as well as your back straight, as well as your hands on your hips.
- Gently raise your knee, as if you are doing knee lifts, but keep it in place for 15 to 60 seconds.
- Rep each leg three times.

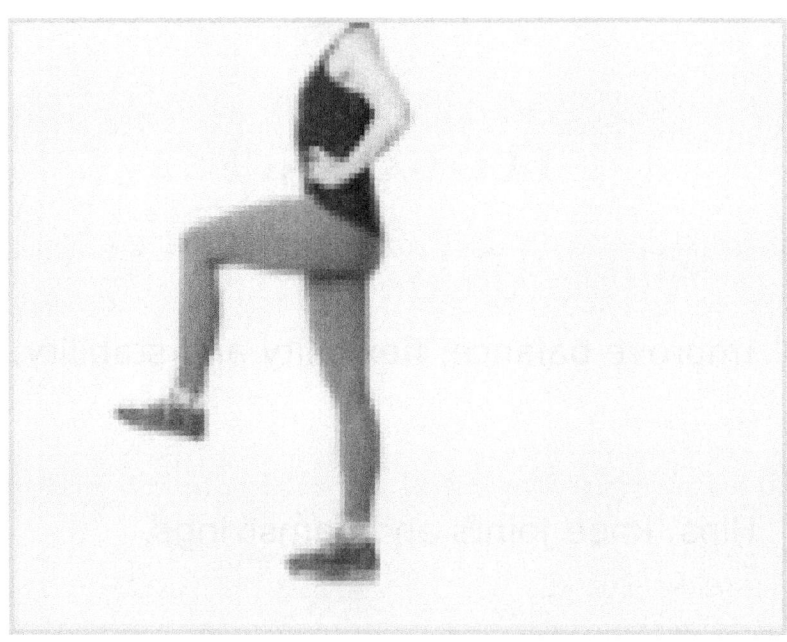

ISOMETRIC CALF RAISE

BENEFIT:

Improve stability, flexibility and balance. Best for injury prevention and rehabilitation.

TARGET:

Target mostly the calves.

PROCEDURE:

- Stand upright with your feet properly separated from each other as well as hold firmly dumbbells in your hands.
- Lift your body from the tip or edge of your front toes while maintaining the rest of your body still.
- Hold the position for up to forty secs. That counts as one rep. Perform three or four sets of ten to

twelve reps, then rest for thirty to sixty seconds before moving on to the next exercise.

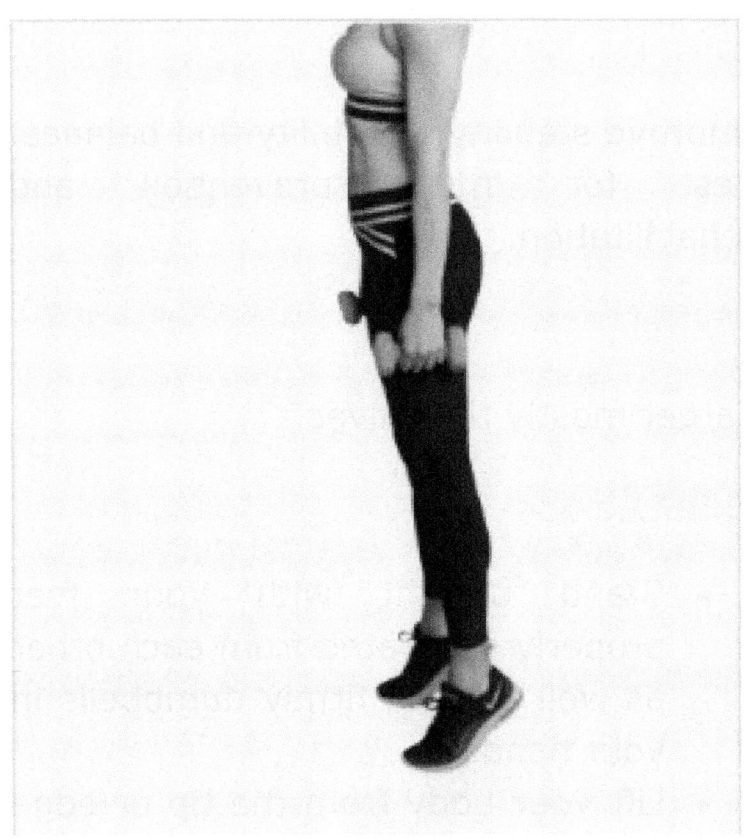

DUCK WALK

BENEFIT:

Strengthen the knee joint, improve balance, range of motion.

TARGET:

Quads and glutes.

PROCEDURE:

- Cross your hands in front of your chest as well as stand with your feet shoulder-width apart.
- Slowly bring down your hips properly into a half squat stance. Lower the right knee first, then the left, while keeping your hips steady.

- Come back to a half-squat by bringing your right foot forward, then your left.
- That counts as one rep. Perform three or four sets of ten to twelve reps on each side, then rest for thirty to sixty seconds before moving on to the next exercise.

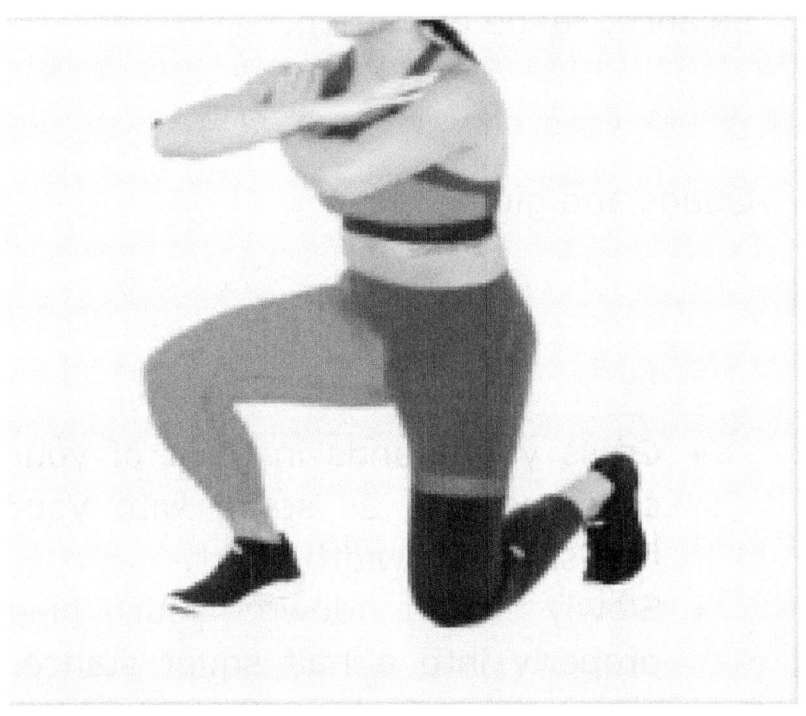

PISTOL SQUAT

BENEFIT:

Strengthen your leg muscles, calves, and joints.

TARGET:

Hips, thighs and quads.

PROCEDURE:

- Begin by placing your feet on the floor.
- Raise your right leg while appropriately maintaining sit on the hips back as well as bending the left knee, lowering the body while maintaining a straight torso.
- For balance, arms can be extended out close to the front chest or out to the sides.

- Return to the beginning point by moving through the left heel that counts as one rep.
- Perform three or four sets of ten to twelve reps on each side, then rest for thirty to sixty seconds.

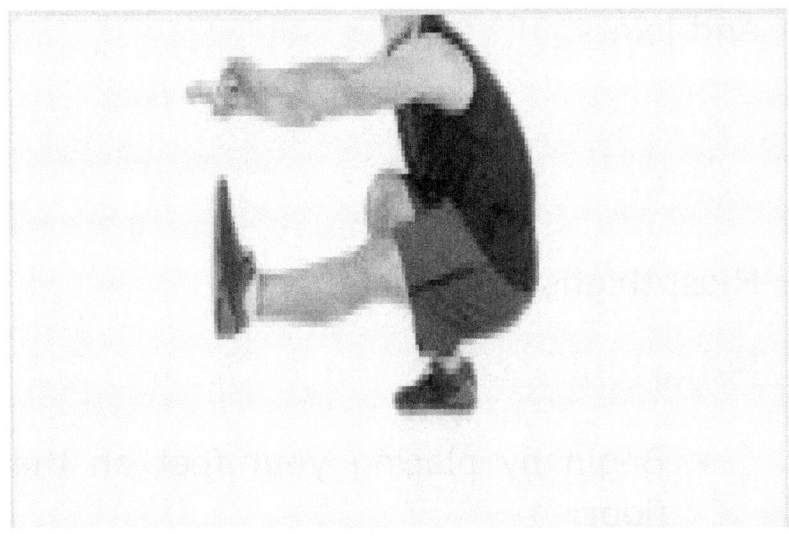

MINI-BAND CLAMSHELLS

BENEFIT:

Strengthen the legs, knee joints and thighs.

TARGET:

Knee joints, glutes and hips.

PROCEDURE:

- Start by lying on your right side properly and ensure that your knees are bent.
- Place a band at your thighs to help to support yourself up and stay solid.
- Position your left hand appropriately on the floor and also ensure that your right arm bend 90-degree.
- Squeeze glutes as well as thigh muscles even against the band to

lift the left thigh then slowly return the left thigh to its original position.
- Perform 4 or 6 sets of ten to twelve reps on each side, then rest for thirty to sixty seconds before moving on to the next exercise.

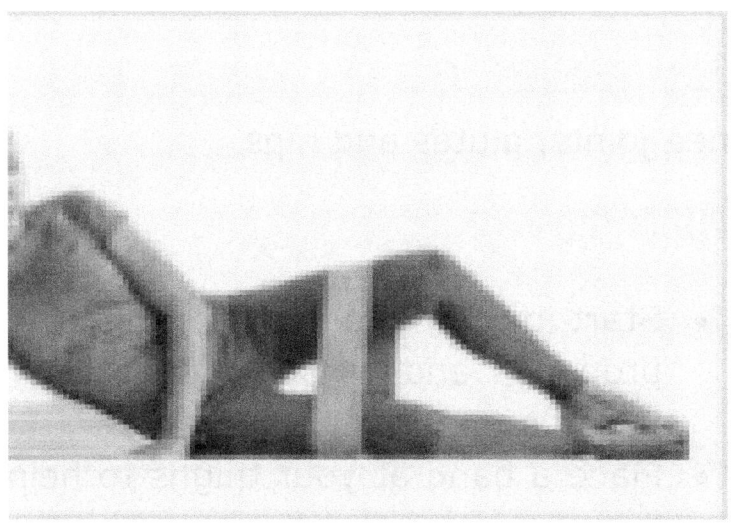

BANDED GLUTE BRIDGE

BENEFIT:

Strengthen the thighs as well as your knee joints.

TARGET:

Thighs, hips and knee joints.

PROCEDURE:

- Start by placing a band at your thigh region and lie down with your back. Your face facing up.
- Raise your back up by bending at least 90 degrees of your outer knee and your feet are placed on the floor.
- Your knees should be above your body level. Your hands should be on the floor flat for support.

- Hold on to the posture and open your legs apart by stretching the band from the knees.
- Return to the beginning. Perform three or four sets of ten to twelve reps, then rest for 30 to 60 seconds before moving on to the next exercise.

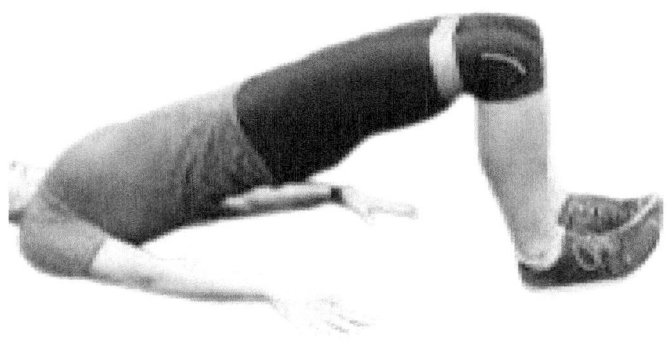

Printed in Great Britain
by Amazon